The Comprehensive KETO Chaffle Cooking Guide

Delicious And Healthy Chaffle Recipes For Beginners

Lily Sherman

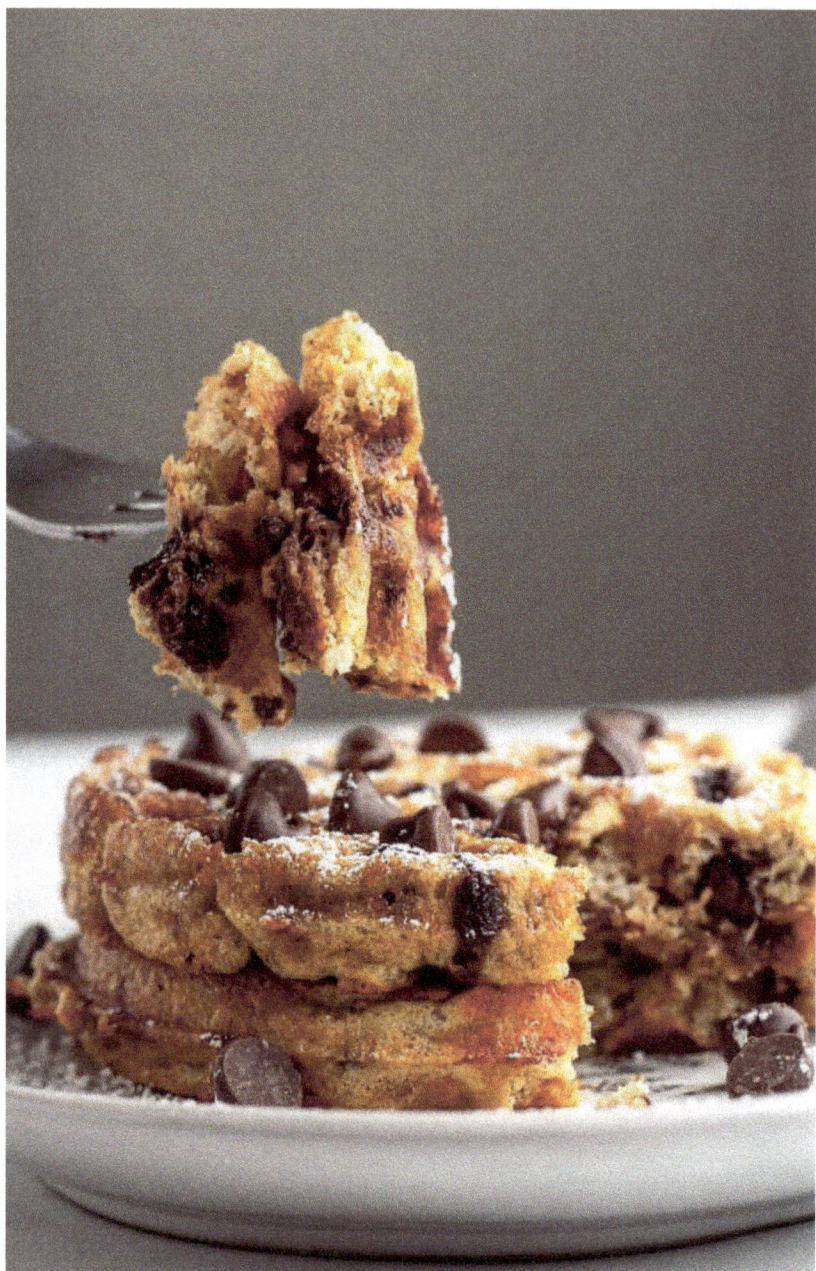

Table of contents

Dairy free Chaffle

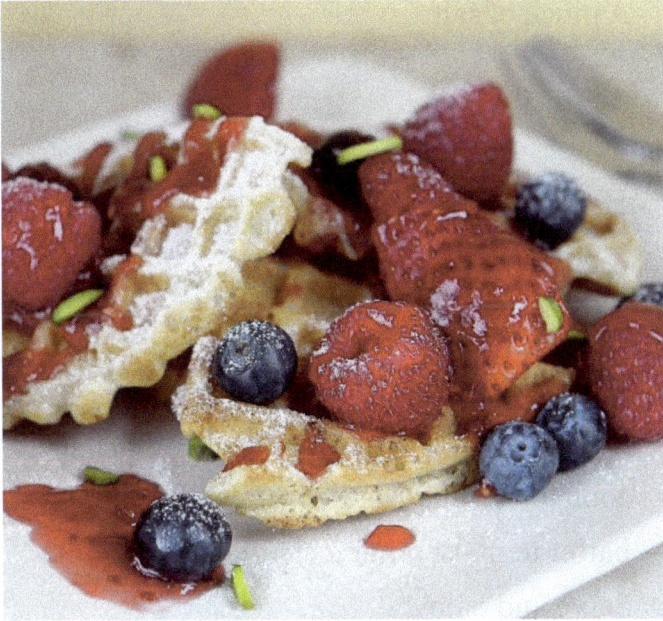

Preparation: 2 minutes

Cooking: 12 minutes

Servings: 3 chaffles

Ingredients

- 1 tbsp coconut flour
- 1 tbsp beef gelatin powder

- 2 eggs
- 1 tbsp mayonnaise
- A pinch of salt

Directions

1. Heat up the mini waffle maker.
2. Mix now the coconut flour, beef gelatin and salt in a tiny mixing bowl.
3. Whisk in the eggs and mayonnaise.
4. Pour 1/3 of the batter into your waffle maker and cook for 4 minutes. Repeat now with the rest of the batter to make other 2 chaffles.
5. Serve and enjoy!

Rosemary Chaffles

Cooking: 8 Minutes

Servings: 2

Ingredients

- 1 organic egg, beaten
- 1/2 cup Cheddar cheese, shredded
- 1 tbspn almond flour
- 1 tbspn fresh rosemary, chopped
- Pinch of salt and freshly ground black pepper

Directions

1. Preheat now a mini waffle iron and then grease it.

For chaffles:

1. In a bowl, place all ingredients and with a fork, Mix well until well combined.
2. Place half of the mixture into Preheat nowed waffle iron and cook for about 4 minutes or until golden brown.
3. Repeat now with the remaining mixture.
4. Serve warm.

Nutrition:

Calories: 173, Net Carb: 11g, Fat: 13.7g, Saturated Fat: 9g, Carbohydrates: 2.29g, Dietary Fiber: 1.1g, Sugar: 0.8g, Protein: 9.99g

White Bread Keto Chaffle | Wonder Bread Chaffle

Preparation: 2 minutes+

Cooking: 8 minutes

Servings: 2

Ingredients

- 1 Egg
- 3 tbsp Almond Flour
- 1 tbsp Mayonnaise
- 1/4 tsp Baking Powder
- 1 tsp Water

Directions

1. Preheat now mini waffle maker.
2. In a bowl, whisk the egg until beaten.
3. Add almond flour, mayonnaise, baking powder, and water.
4. When your waffle maker is heated, carefully pour 1/2 of the batter in your waffle maker and close the top. Allow to cook for 3-5 minutes.

5. Carefully Remove now from your waffle maker and set aside for 2-3 minutes to crisp up.

6. Do it again for the second chaffle.

Nutrition:

Calories: 125, Total Fat: 11.5g, Carbohydrates: 2g, Fiber: 1g, Protein: 5g

Keto Rye Bread Chaffle

Preparation: 15-20 minutes

Servings: 1

Ingredients

- 1 egg
- 2 tbsps almond flour
- 1 tbspn Melt nowed butter
- 1 tbspn mozzarella cheese
- pinch salt
- pinch garlic powder
- 1/2 teaspn baking powder
- 1/2 teaspn caraway seeds

Directions

1. Preheat now mini waffle maker.
2. Mix all rye bread chaffle ingredients in a tiny bowl.
3. Place 1/2 the mixture into a Preheat nowed mini waffle maker.
4. Cook for 4 minutes.
5. Serve warm.

Nutrition:

Calories: 263kcal, Carbohydrates: 3.1g, Protein: 10.6g, Fat: 18.8g, Fiber: 0.6g , Sugar: 0.8g,

Chaffle Churros

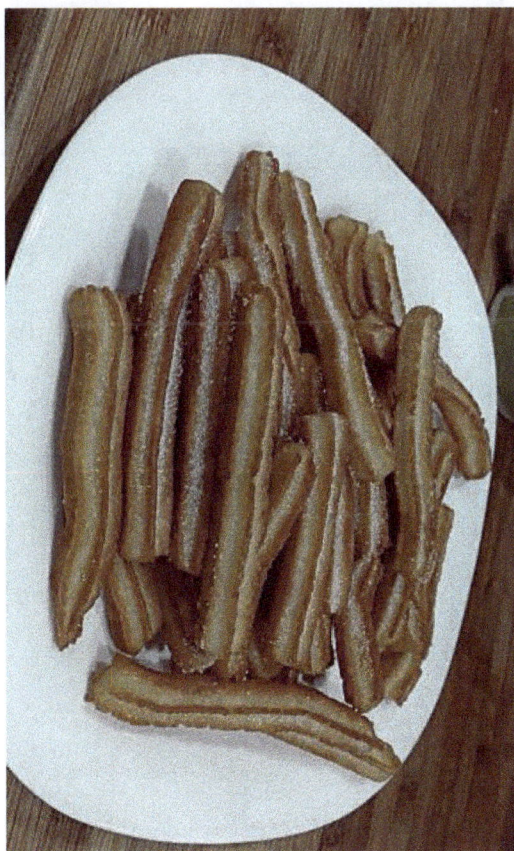

Preparation: 10 min.

Cooking: 5 min.

Servings: 2

Ingredients

- 1 egg
- 1 Tbsp. almond flour
- ½ tsp. vanilla extract
- 1 tsp. cinnamon, divided
- ¼ tsp. baking powder
- ½ cup shredded mozzarella
- 1 Tbsp. swerve confectioners' sugar substitute
- 1 Tbsp. swerve brown sugar substitute
- 1 Tbsp. butter, Melt nowed

Directions

1. Turn on waffle maker to heat and oil it with cooking spray.
2. Mix egg, flour, vanilla extract, ½ tsp. cinnamon, baking powder, mozzarella, and sugar substitute in a bowl.
3. Place half of the mixture into waffle maker and cooking for 3-5 min, or until desired doneness. Remove now and place the second half of the batter into the maker.
4. Cut chaffles into strips.
5. Place strips in a bowl and cover with Melt nowed butter.

6. Mix brown sugar substitute and the remaining cinnamon in a bowl. Pour sugar mixture over the strips and toss to coat them well.

Nutrition:

Calories: 372, Fat: 16g, Carbs: 3g, Protein: 40g.

Cocoa Chaffles

Preparation: 5 min.

Cooking: 5 min.

Servings: 2

Ingredients

- 1 egg
- 1½ Tbsp. unsweetened cocoa
- 2 Tbsp. lakanto monk fruit, or choice of sweetener
- 1 Tbsp. heavy cream
- 1 tsp. coconut flour
- ½ tsp. baking powder
- ½ tsp. vanilla

For the Cheese Cream:

- 1 Tbsp. lakanto powdered sweetener
- 2 Tbsp. softened cream cheese
- ¼ tsp. vanilla

Directions

1. Turn on waffle maker to heat and oil it with cooking spray. Combine all chaffle ingredients in a tiny bowl.
2. Pour one half of the chaffle mixture into waffle maker. Cooking for 3-5 minutes.
3. Remove now and Repeat now with the second half if the mixture. Let chaffles sit for 2-3 to crisp up.
4. Combine all cream ingredients and spread on chaffle when they have cooled to room temperature.

Nutrition:

Calories: 343g. Fat: 27g, Carbs: 4g, Protein: 21g

Fresh Dill Chaffle

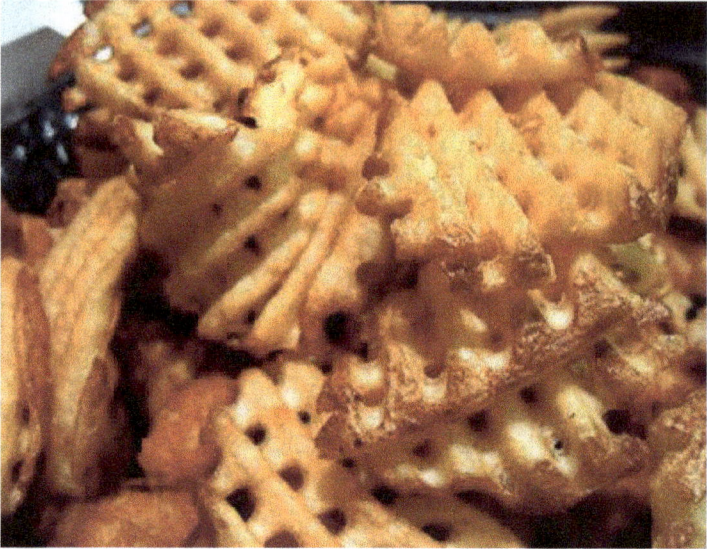

Preparation: 5 minutes

Cooking: 8 minutes

Servings: 2 chaffles

Ingredients

- 1 egg, beaten
- ½ cup shredded cheddar cheese
- ½ tbsp fresh dill, finely chopped

Directions

1. Heat up your waffle maker.

2. Add egg, shredded cheddar cheese, and dill to a tiny mixing bowl and combine well.

3. Pour half of the batter into your waffle maker and cook for 4 minutes until brown. Repeat now with the rest of the batter to make another chaffle.

4. Serve with your favorite keto dressing and enjoy!

Italian Bread Chaffle

Preparation: 15 minutes

Cooking: 20 minutes

Servings: 2

Ingredients

For the Chaffle:

- Egg: 2
- Mozzarella cheese: 1 cup (shredded)
- Garlic powder: ½ tsp.
- Italian seasoning: 1 tsp.
- Cream cheese: 1 tsp.

For the Garlic Butter Topping:

- Garlic powder: ½ tsp.
- Italian seasoning: ½ tsp.
- Butter: 1 tbsp.

For Cheesy Bread:

- Mozzarella cheese: 2 tbsp. (shredded)
- Parsley: 1 tbsp.

Directions

1. Preheat now a mini waffle maker if needed and grease it
2. In a mixing bowl, add all the ingredients of the chaffle and mix well
3. Pour the mixture to the lower plate of your waffle maker and spread it evenly to cover the plate properly and close the lid
4. Cooking for at least 4 minutes to get the desired crunch
5. In the meanwhile, melt now butter and add the garlic butter ingredients
6. Remove now the chaffle from the heat and apply the garlic butter immediately
7. Make as many chaffles as your mixture and waffle maker allow
8. Put the chaffles on the baking tray and sprinkle the Mozzarella cheese on the chaffles
9. Bake for 5 minutes in an oven at 350 degrees to Melt now the cheese
10. Serve hot and enjoy.

Nutrition:

Calories: 181; Total Fat: 19g; Carbs: 4g; Net Carbs: 2g; Fiber: 2g; Protein: 1g

Fresh Coriander Chaffle

Preparation: 5 minutes

Cooking: 8 minutes

Servings: 2 chaffles

Ingredients

- 1 egg, beaten
- ½ cup shredded mozzarella cheese
- 1 tsp coconut flour
- ¼ tsp baking powder
- ½ tsp fresh coriander, minced

Directions

1. Heat up your waffle maker.
2. Add all the ingredients to a tiny mixing bowl and combine well.
3. Pour half of the batter into your waffle maker and cook for 4 minutes until golden brown. Repeat now with the rest of the batter to make another chaffle.
4. Let cool for 3 minutes to let chaffles get crispy.
5. Serve and enjoy!

Cornbread Chaffle

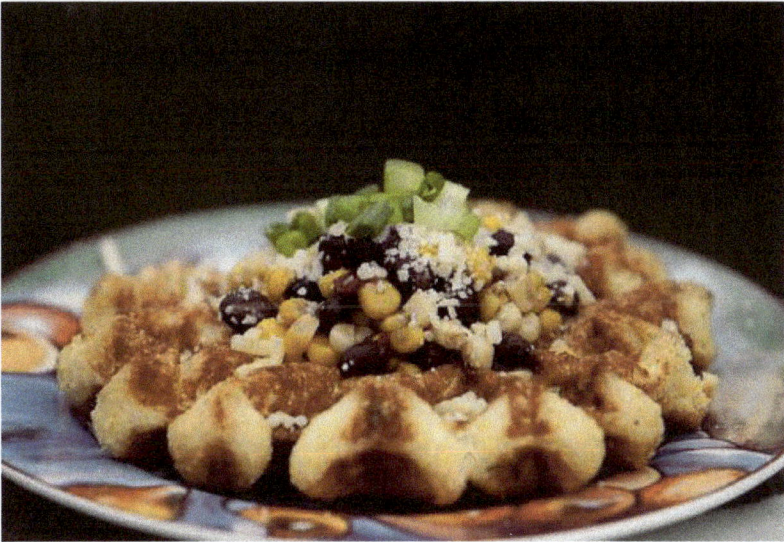

Preparation: 5 minutes

Cooking: 8 minutes

Servings: 2 chaffles

Ingredients

- 1 egg, beaten
- ½ cup shredded cheddar cheese
- ¼ tsp corn bread extract
- ¼ tsp baking powder

25

- A pinch of salt and pepper

Directions

1. Heat up your waffle maker.
2. Add all the ingredients to a tiny mixing bowl and stir until well combined.
3. Pour half of the batter into your waffle maker and cook for 4 minutes until brown. Repeat now with the rest of the batter to make another chaffle.
4. Let cool for 3 minutes to let chaffles get crispy.
5. Serve and enjoy!

Soft Chaffle

Preparation: 5 minutes

Cooking: 16 minutes

Servings: 4 chaffles

Ingredients

- ¼ cup almond flour
- ½ cup mozzarella cheese, shredded
- 1 egg, beaten
- 1 large egg white
- 2 tbsp cream cheese
- 1 tbsp sweetener
- ½ tsp baking powder
- ¼ tsp vanilla extract
- 2 tbsp coconut flour

Directions

1. Heat up the mini waffle maker.
2. Add all the ingredients to a tiny mixing bowl and combine well.

3. Pour ¼ of the batter into your waffle maker and cook for 4 minutes until golden brown. Then cook the remaining batter to prepare the other chaffles.
4. Serve and enjoy!

Savory Chaffle

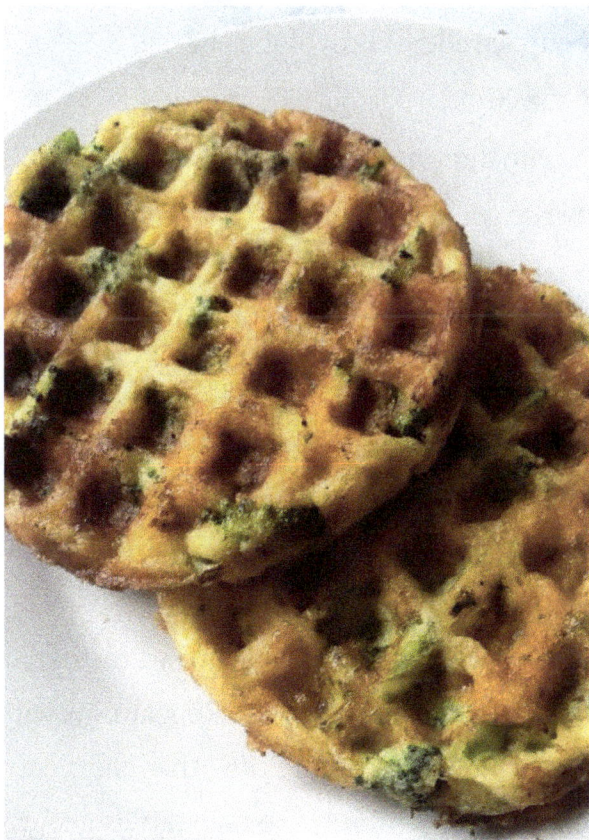

Preparation: 5 minutes

Cooking: 16 minutes

Servings: 4 chaffles

Ingredients

- 4 eggs, beaten
- 1 cup shredded Provolone cheese
- 1 cup Mozzarella cheese, shredded
- ½ cup almond flour
- 2 tbsp coconut flour
- 2 tsp baking powder
- A pinch of salt and pepper

Directions

1. Heat up your waffle maker.
2. Add all the ingredients to a tiny mixing bowl and combine well.
3. Pour ¼ of the batter into your waffle maker and cook for 4 minutes until brown. Repeat now with the rest of the batter to prepare the other chaffles.
4. Let cool for 3 minutes to let chaffles get crispy.
5. Serve and enjoy!

Egg-free Chaffle

Preparation: 5 minutes

Cooking: 4 minutes

Servings: 1 chaffle

Ingredients

- 2 tbsp mozzarella cheese, shredded
- 1 tbsp cream cheese
- 1 tbsp psyllium husk powder

Directions

1. Heat up your waffle maker.
2. Add all the ingredients to a tiny mixing bowl and combine well.
3. Pour the batter into your waffle maker and cook for 4 minutes until brown.
4. Let cool for 3 minutes to let chaffles get crispy.
5. Serve and enjoy!

Traditional Chaffle

Preparation: 5 minutes

Cooking: 8 minutes

Servings: 2 chaffles

Ingredients

- 1 egg, beaten
- ½ cup of mozzarella cheese, shredded
- 2 tbsp almond flour
- ¼ tsp baking powder
- ½ psyllium husk powder

Directions

1. Heat up your waffle maker.
2. Add all the ingredients to a tiny mixing bowl and stir until well combined.
3. Pour half of the batter into your waffle maker and cook for 4 minutes until golden brown. Repeat now with the rest of the batter to make another chaffle.
4. Let cool for 3 minutes to let chaffles get crispy.
5. Serve and enjoy!

Curry Chaffle

Preparation: 5 minutes

Cooking: 8 minutes

Servings: 2 chaffles

Ingredients

- 1 egg, beaten
- ½ cup shredded mozzarella cheese
- ½ tsp curry powder
- ½ tsp fresh basil, finely chopped

Directions

1. Heat up your waffle maker.
2. Add egg, shredded mozzarella cheese, curry powder and basil to a tiny mixing bowl and combine well.
3. Pour half of the batter into your waffle maker and cook for 4 minutes until brown. Repeat now with the rest of the batter to make another chaffle.
4. Serve and enjoy!

Blue Cheese Chaffle

Preparation: 5 minutes

Cooking: 8 minutes

Servings: 2 chaffles

Ingredients

- 1 large egg, beaten
- ½ cup Blue cheese, shredded
- 1 tsp sweetener

Directions

1. Heat up your waffle maker.
2. Add all the ingredients to a tiny mixing bowl and stir until well combined.
3. Pour half of the batter into your waffle maker and cook for 4 minutes until golden brown. Repeat now with the rest of the batter to make another chaffle.
4. Let cool for 3 minutes to let chaffles get crispy.
5. Serve and enjoy!

Chives Chaffle

Preparation: 5 minutes

Cooking: 8 minutes

Servings: 2 chaffles

Ingredients

- 1 large egg, beaten
- ½ cup of mozzarella cheese, shredded
- 2 tbsp almond flour
- ¼ tsp baking powder
- 1 tbsp chopped fresh chives

Directions

1. Heat up your waffle maker.
2. Add all the ingredients to a tiny mixing bowl and combine well.
3. Pour half of the batter into your waffle maker and cook for 4 minutes until brown. Repeat now with the rest of the batter to make another chaffle.
4. Let cool for 3 minutes to let chaffles get crispy.
5. Serve and enjoy!

Ricotta Chaffle

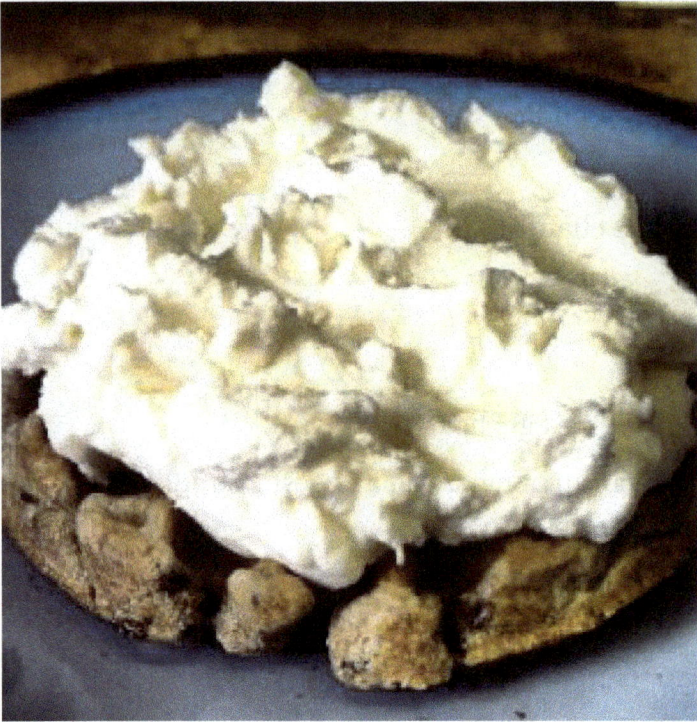

Preparation: 5 minutes

Cooking: 8 minutes

Servings: 2 chaffles

Ingredients

- 1 large egg, beaten

- ½ cup skim ricotta cheese
- 2 tbsp almond flour
- ½ tsp baking powder

Directions

1. Heat up your waffle maker.
2. Add all the ingredients to a tiny mixing bowl and stir until well combined.
3. Pour half of the batter into your waffle maker and cook for 4 minutes until golden brown. Repeat now with the rest of the batter to make another chaffle.
4. Let cool for 3 minutes to let chaffles get crispy.
5. Serve and enjoy!

Mini Breakfast Chaffles

Cooking: 15 Minutes

Servings: 3

Ingredients

- 6 tsp coconut flour
- 1 tsp stevia
- 1/4 tsp baking powder
- 2 eggs
- 3 oz. cream cheese
- 1/2. tsp vanilla extract

<u>Topping:</u>

- 1 egg
- 6 slice bacon
- 2 oz. Raspberries for topping
- 2 oz. Blueberries for topping
- 2 oz. Strawberries for topping

Directions

1. Heat up your square waffle maker and grease with cooking spray.

2. Mix coconut flour, stevia, egg, baking powder, cheese and vanilla in mixing bowl.
3. Pour ½ of chaffles mixture in a waffle maker.
4. Close the lid and cook the chaffles for about 3-5 minutesutes.
5. Meanwhile, fry bacon slices in pan on medium heat for about 2-3 minutes until cooked and transfer them to plate.
6. In the same pan, fry eggs one by one in the bacon's leftover grease.
7. Once chaffles are cooked, carefully transfer them to a plate.
8. Serve with fried eggs and bacon slice and berries on top.
9. Enjoy!

Nutrition:

Protein: 16% 75 kcal, Fat: 75% 346 kcal, Carbohydrates: 9% 41 kcal

Crispy Chaffles With Egg & Asparagus

Cooking: 10 Minutes

Servings: 1

Ingredients

- 1 egg
- 1/4 cup cheddar cheese
- 2 tbsps. almond flour
- ½ tsp. baking powder

Topping:

- 1 egg
- 4-5 stalks asparagus
- 1 tsp avocado oil

Directions

1. Preheat now waffle maker to medium-high heat.
2. Whisk together egg, mozzarella cheese, almond flour, and baking powder
3. Pour chaffles mixture into the center of the waffle iron. Close your waffle maker and cook for 5 minute or until the waffle is golden brown and set.

4. Remove now chaffles from your waffle maker and serve.
5. Meanwhile, heat oil in a nonstick pan.
6. Once the pan is hot, fry asparagus for about 4-5 minutes until golden brown.
7. Poach the egg in boil water for about 2-3 minutes.
8. Once chaffles are cooked, Remove now from the maker.
9. Serve chaffles with the poached egg and asparagus.

Nutrition:

Protein: 26% 85 kcal, Fat: 69% 226 kcal, Carbohydrates: 5% 16 kcal

Cheese Chaffle Recipe with Cinnamon, Vanilla & Almond Flour

Preparation: 10 minutes

Cooking: 5 minutes

Servings: 2

Ingredients

- 1 egg
- 115 g grated mozzarella
- 1 tbsp almond flour
- 1 teaspn Baking powder
- 1 tsp vanilla extract
- 1 pinch of cinnamon Fat for the chaffle maker

Directions:

1. Mix now the egg with the vanilla extract.
2. Mix now the dry ingredients in a separate bowl and add them to the egg.
3. Finally, fold in the cheese, grease the chaffle iron and pour half of the dough into it.
4. Now bake the chaffle for about 5 minutes or until it is golden brown and crispy.

5. Check periodically so that it doesn't burn.

6. Repeat now with the other half of the batter and serve the still warm chaffles with a little butter and low-carb syrup as you like.

Crunch Cereal Cake Chaffle

Preparation: 10 minutes

Cooking: 5 minutes

Servings: 1

Ingredients

For the chaffles:

- 1 egg
- 2 tbsp. almond flour
- 1/2 tsp. coconut flour
- 1 tbsp. butter, Melt nowed
- 1 tbsp. cream cheese, softened
- 1/4 tsp. vanilla extract
- 1/4 tsp. baking powder
- 1 tbsp. confectioners' sweetener
- 1/8 tsp. xanthan gum

For the toppings:

- 20 drops captain cereal flavoring
- Whipped cream

Directions:

1. Preheat now the mini waffle maker.
2. Blend or mix all the chaffles ingredients until the consistency is creamy and smooth. Allow to rest for a few minutes so that the flour absorbs the liquid ingredients.
3. Scoop out 2-3 tbsp. of batter and put it into your waffle maker. Allow to cooking for 2-3 minutes.
4. Top the cooked chaffles with freshly whipped cream.
5. Add syrup and drops of Captain Cereal flavoring for a great flavor.

Nutrition:

36.4g Protein, 10.4g Carbohydrates, 7.7g Fat, 2g Fiber, 101mg Cholesterol, 99mg Sodium, 697mg Potassium.

Keto Chaffle Breakfast Sandwich

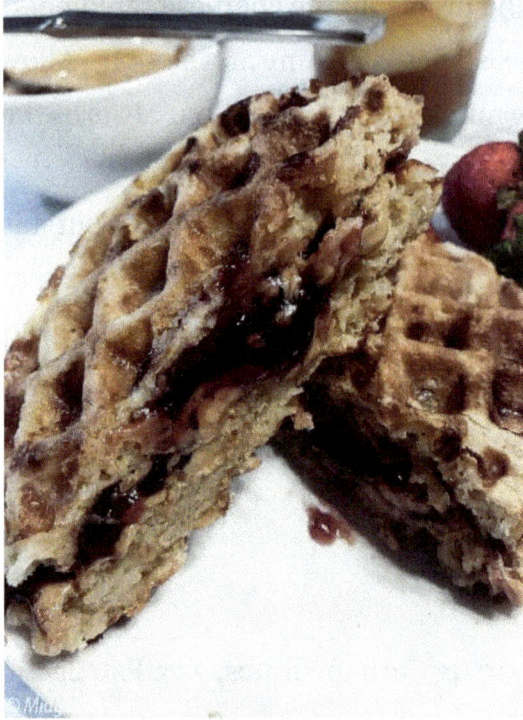

Preparation: 3 minutes

Cooking: 6 minutes

Servings: 1

Ingredients

- 1 egg
- 1/2 cup Monterey Jack Cheese

- 1 tbspn almond flour
- 2 tbsps butter

Directions

1. In a tiny bowl, mix now the egg, almond flour, and Monterey Jack Cheese.
2. Pour half of the batter into your mini waffle maker and cooking for 3-4 minutes. Then cooking the rest of the batter to make a second chaffle.
3. In a tiny pan, Melt now 2 tbsps of butter. Add the chaffles and cooking on each side for 2 minutes. Pressing down while they are cooking lightly on the top of them, so they crisp up better.
4. Remove now from the pan and let sit for 2 minutes.

Nutrition:

Calories: 312, Fat: 19g, Carbs: 4,8, Protein: 22g.

Keto Chaffle Taco Shells

Preparation: 5 minutes

Cooking: 20 minutes

Servings: 5

Ingredients

- 1 tbspn almond flour
- 1 cup taco blend cheese
- 2 eggs
- 1/4 tsp. taco seasoning

Directions

1. In a bowl, mix almond flour, taco blend cheese, eggs, and taco seasoning. I find it easiest to mix everything using a fork.
2. Add 1.5 tbsps of taco chaffle batter to your waffle maker at a time — Cooking chaffle batter in your waffle maker for 4 minutes.
3. Remove now the taco chaffle shell from your waffle maker and drape over the side of a bowl. I used my

pie pan because it was what I had on hand, but just about any bowl will work.

4. Continue making chaffle taco shells until you are out of batter. Then fill your taco shells with taco meat, your favorite toppings, and enjoy!

Nutrition:

Calories: 476, Fat: 18g, Carbs: 8g, Protein: 21g.

French Dip Chaffle Sandwich

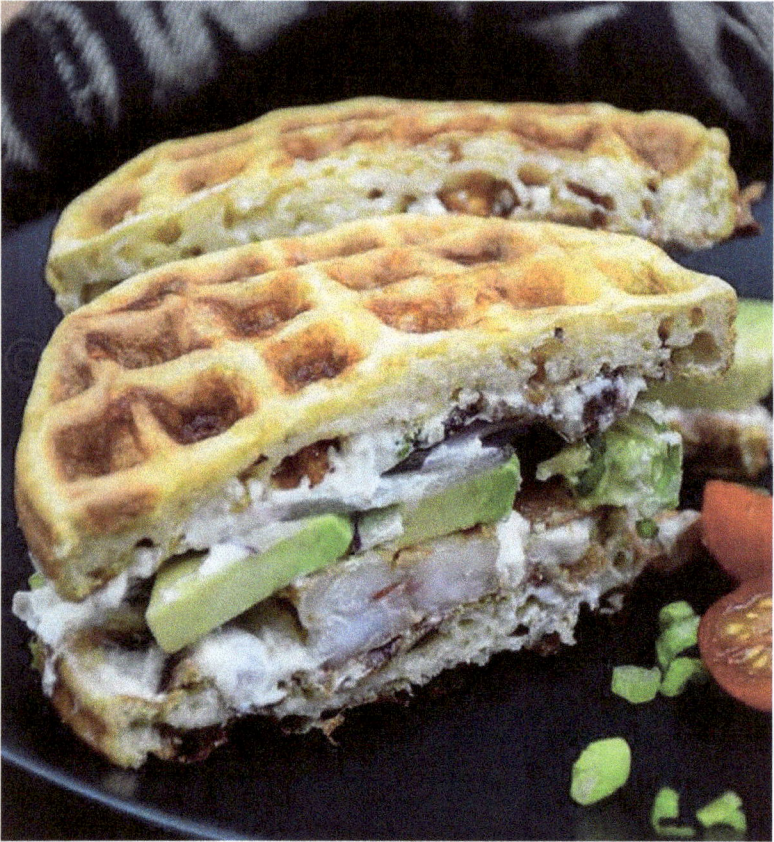

Preparation: 5 minutes

Cooking: 12 minutes

Servings: 2

Ingredients

- 1 egg white
- 1/4 cup Mozzarella cheese, shredded (packed)
- 1/4 cup sharp cheddar cheese, shredded (packed) 3/4 tsp. water
- 1 tsp. coconut flour
- 1/4 tsp. baking powder
- Pinch of salt

Directions

1. Preheat now oven to 425 degrees. Plug the Dash Mini Waffle Maker in the wall and grease lightly once it is hot.
2. Combine all of the ingredients in a bowl and stir to combine.
3. Spoon out 1/2 of the batter on your waffle maker and close lid. Set a timer for 4 minutes and do not lift the lid until the cooking time is complete. Lifting beforehand can cause the Chaffle keto sandwich recipe to separate and stick to the waffle iron. You have to let it cooking the entire 4 minutes before lifting the lid.

4. Remove now the chaffle from the waffle iron and set aside. Repeat the same steps above with the rest of the chaffle batter.

5. Cover a cooking sheet with parchment paper and place chaffles a few inches apart.

6. Add 1/4 to 1/3 cup of of the slow cooker keto roast beef from the following recipe. Make sure to drain the excess broth/gravy before adding to the top of the chaffle.

7. Add a slice of deli cheese or shredded cheese on top. Swiss and provolone are both great options. Place on the top rack of the oven for 5 minutes so that the cheese can Melt now. If you'd like the cheese to bubble and begin to brown, turn oven to broil for 1 min. (The swiss cheese may not brown) Enjoy open-faced with a tiny bowl of beef broth for dipping.

Nutrition:

Calories: 510, Fat: 35g, Carbs: 2g, Protein: 44g.

Bacon & Cheddar Cheese Chaffles

Preparation: 5 minutes

Cooking: 5 minutes

Servings: 6

Ingredients

- ½ cup almond flour
- 3 bacon strips
- ¼ cup sour cream
- 1 ½ cup cheddar cheese
- ½ cup smoked Gouda cheese
- ½ tsp. onion powder
- ½ tsp. baking powder
- ¼ cup oat
- 1 egg
- 1 tbsp. oil
- 1 ½ tbsp. butter
- ¼ tsp. salt
- ½ tsp. parsley
- ¼ tsp. baking soda

Directions

1. Heat your waffle maker.
2. Take a bowl add almond flour, baking powder, baking soda, onion powder, garlic salt and mix well.
3. In another bowl whisk eggs, bacon, cream, parsley, butter and cheese until well combined.
4. Now pour the mixture over dry ingredients and mix well.
5. Pour the batter over the Preheat nowed waffle maker and cooking for 5 to 6 minutes or until golden brown.
6. Serve the hot and crispy chaffles.

Nutrition:

Net Carbs: 1.2g; Calories: 233.6; Total Fat: 11.7g; Saturated Fat: 1.3g; Protein: 30.9g; Carbs: 1.2g; Fiber: 0g; Sugar: 0g

Jalapeno & Bacon Chaffle

Preparation: 5 minutes

Cooking: 5 minutes

Servings: 6

Ingredients

- 3 tbsp. coconut flour
- 1 tsp. baking powder
- 3 eggs
- 8 oz. cream cheese
- ¼ tsp. salt
- 4 bacon slices
- 2 to 3 jalapenos
- 1 cup cheddar cheese

Directions

1. Wash the jalapeno and slice them.
2. Take a pan and cooking jalapeno until golden brown or crispy.
3. Take a bowl add flour, baking powder and salt and mix.
4. In a mixing bowl add cream and beat well until fluffy.

5. Now in another bowl add egg and whisk them well.
6. Pour cream, cheese and beat until well combined.
7. Add the mixture with dry ingredients and make a smooth batter. After that fold the jalapeno in mixture.
8. Heat your waffle maker and pour the batter into it.
9. Cooking it for 5 minutes or until golden brown.
10. Top it with cheese, jalapeno and crème and serve the hot chaffles.

Nutrition:

Net Carbs: 2.8g; Calories: 310; Total Fat: 20g; Saturated Fat: 4.8g; Protein: 30.2g; Carbs: 3.1g; Fiber: 0.3g; Sugar: 1.2g

Breakfast Chaffle Sandwich

Preparation: 30 mins

Cooking: 5 mins

Ingredients

- 1 egg
- ½ cup of shredded mozzarella cheese
- 2 Tbspn of coconut flour
- ½ tsp of baking powder
- 1 teaspn of Italian herbs
- 2 tbspn of almond oil
- 2 slices of tomato
- 2 slices of lettuce

Directions

1. Take shredded mozzarella, egg, baking powder, Italian herbs and mix now them well in a bowl.
2. Then turn on your waffle machine to medium heat. Pour the batter in the waffle machine.
3. Don't open the machine before 3 minutes and let it cook until it is golden brown.

4. Now you can take a pan and turn on the heat to medium. Then add the unsalted butter in the pan and let it Melt now.
5. Once the butter Melt nows, add chaffle and cook it in the butter until it becomes crispy.
6. Make sure you cook both sides well. Then assemble your sandwich. Add your vegetables in the sandwich and enjoy your healthy and nutritious breakfast.

Nutrition:

Calories 514, Fat 32g, Protein 22g, Carbohydrates 3g

Coconut Chaffles

Cooking: 5 Minutes

Servings: 2

Ingredients

- 1 egg
- 1 oz. cream cheese,
- 1 oz. cheddar cheese
- 2 tbsps. coconut flour
- 1 tsp. stevia
- 1 tbsp. coconut oil, Melt nowed
- 1/2 tsp. coconut extract
- 2 eggs, soft boil for serving

Directions

1. Heat you waffle maker and grease with cooking spray.
2. Mix all chaffles ingredients in a bowl.
3. Pour chaffle batter in a Preheat nowed waffle maker.
4. Close the lid.
5. Cook chaffles for about 2-3 minutesutes until golden brown.

6. Serve with boil egg and enjoy!

Nutrition:

Protein: 21% 32 kcal, Fat: % 117 kcal, Carbohydrates: 3% 4 kcal

Scrambled Eggs on A Spring Onion Chaffle

Cooking: 7–9 Minutes

Servings: 4

Ingredients

<u>Batter:</u>

- 4 eggs
- 2 cups grated mozzarella cheese
- 2 spring onions, finely chopped
- Salt and pepper to taste
- ½ teaspn dried garlic powder
- 2 tbsps almond flour
- 2 tbsps coconut flour

<u>Other:</u>

- 2 tbsps butter for brushing your waffle maker
- 6-8 eggs
- Salt and pepper
- 1 teaspn Italian spice mix
- 1 tbspn olive oil
- 1 tbspn freshly chopped parsley

Directions

1. Preheat now your waffle maker.
2. Crack the eggs into a bowl and add the grated cheese.
3. Mix well until just combined, then add the chopped spring onions and season with salt and pepper and dried garlic powder.
4. Stir in the almond flour and Mix well until everything is combined.
5. Brush the heated waffle maker with butter and add a few tbsps of the batter.
6. Close the lid and cook for about 7–8 minutes depending on your waffle maker.
7. While the chaffles are cooking, prepare the scrambled eggs by whisking the eggs in a bowl until frothy, about 2 minutes. Season with salt and black pepper to taste and add the Italian spice mix. Whisk to blend in the spices.
8. Warm the oil in a non-stick pan over medium heat.
9. Pour the eggs in the pan and cook until eggs are set to your liking.
10. Serve each chaffle and top with some scrambled eggs. Top with freshly chopped parsley.

Nutrition:

Calories 194, fat 14.7 g, carbs 5 g, sugar 0.6 g, Protein 1 g, sodium 191 mg

Chaffles Breakfast Bowl

Cooking: 5 Minutes

Servings: 2

Ingredients

Chaffle:

- 1 egg
- 1/2 cup cheddar cheese shredded
- pinch of Italian seasoning
- 1 tbsp. pizza sauce

Topping:

- 1/2 avocado sliced
- 2 eggs boiled
- 1 tomato, halves
- 4 oz. fresh spinach leaves

Directions

1. Preheat now your waffle maker and grease with cooking spray.
2. Crack an egg in a tiny bowl and beat with Italian seasoning and pizza sauce.

3. Add shredded cheese to the egg and spices mixture.
4. Pour 1 tbsp. shredded cheese in a waffle maker and cook for 30 sec.
5. Pour Chaffles batter in your waffle maker and close the lid.
6. Cook chaffles for about 4 minutes until crispy and brown.
7. Carefully Remove now chaffles from the maker.
8. Serve on the spinach bed with boil egg, avocado slice, and tomatoes.
9. Enjoy!

Nutrition:

Protein: 23% 77 kcal, Fat: 66% 222 kcal, Carbohydrates: 11% 39 kcal

Coffee Flavored Chaffle

Preparation: 10 minutes

Cooking: 7–9 Minutes

Servings: 4

Ingredients

Batter:

- 4 eggs
- 4 ounce of cream cheese
- ½ teaspn vanilla extract
- 6 tbsps strong boiled espresso
- ¼ cup stevia
- ½ cup almond flour
- 1 teaspn baking powder
- Pinch of salt

Other:

- 2 tbsps butter to brush your waffle maker

Directions

1. Preheat now your waffle maker.

2. Add the eggs and cream cheese to a bowl and stir in the vanilla extract, espresso, stevia, almond flour, baking powder, and salt pinch.
3. Stir just until everything is combined and fully incorporated.
4. Brush the heated waffle maker with butter and add a few tbsps of the batter.
5. Close the lid and cooking for about 7–8 minutes depending on your waffle maker.
6. Serve and enjoy.

Nutrition:

Kcal 571, Fat 45g, Net Carbs 8.2g, Protein 41g

Japanese Breakfast Chaffle

Cooking: 10 Minutes

Servings: 2

Ingredients

- 1 egg
- 1/2 cup shredded mozzarella cheese
- 1 Tbsp Kewpie mayo
- 1 stalk of green onion, chopped
- 1 slice bacon, chopped

Directions

1. Turn on your waffle maker to heat and oil with cooking spray
2. Beat egg in tiny bowl
3. Add 1 Tbsp mayo, bacon, and 1/2 green. Mix well
4. 4 Place 1/3 cup of of cheese on waffle maker, then spread half of the egg mixture over it and top with 1/3 cup of cheese.
5. Close and cook for 3-4 minutes
6. Repeat for the remaining batter

7. Transfer to a plate and sprinkle with remaining green onion.

Nutrition:

Carbs: 1 g, Fat: 16 g, Calories: 183

Morning Chaffles With Berries

Cooking: 5 Minutes

Servings: 4

Ingredients

- 1 cup egg whites
- 1 cup cheddar cheese, shredded
- ¼ cup almond flour
- ¼ cup heavy cream

Topping:

- 4 oz. raspberries
- 4 oz. strawberries.
- 1 oz. keto chocolate flakes
- 1 oz. feta cheese.

Directions

1. Preheat now your square waffle maker and grease with cooking spray.
2. Beat egg white in a tiny bowl with flour.
3. Add shredded cheese to the egg whites and flour mixture and mix well.

4. Add cream and cheese to the egg mixture.

5. Pour Chaffles batter in a waffle maker and close the lid.

6. Cook chaffles for about 4 minutes until crispy and brown.

7. Carefully Remove now chaffles from the maker.

8. Serve with berries, cheese, and chocolate on top.

9. Enjoy!

Nutrition:

Protein: 28% 68 kcal, Fat: 67% 163 kcal, Carbohydrates: 5% 12 kcal

Raspberry-Yogurt Chaffle Bowl

Preparation: 10 minutes

Cooking: 14 minutes

Servings: 2

Ingredients

- 1 egg, beaten
- 1 tbsp almond flour
- ¼ cup finely grated mozzarella cheese
- ¼ tsp baking powder
- 1 cup Greek yogurt
- 1 cup fresh raspberries
- 2 tbsp almonds, chopped

Directions

1. Preheat now a waffle bowl maker and grease lightly with cooking spray.
2. Meanwhile, in a bowl, whisk all the ingredients except the yogurt, raspberries until smooth batter forms.

3. Open the iron, pour in half of the mixture, cover, and cook until crispy, 6 to 7 minutes.

4. Remove now the chaffle bowl onto a plate and set aside.

5. Make the second chaffle bowl with the remaining batter.

6. To serve, divide the yogurt into the chaffle bowls and top with the raspberries and almonds.

Bacon-Cheddar Biscuit Chaffle

Preparation: 10 minutes

Cooking: 28 minutes

Servings: 4

Ingredients

- 1 egg, beaten
- 2 tbsp almond flour
- 2 tbsp ground flaxseed
- 3 bacon slices, cooked and chopped
- ¼ cup heavy cream
- 1 ½ tbsp Melt nowed butter
- ½ cup finely grated Gruyere cheese
- ½ cup finely grated cheddar cheese
- ¼ tsp erythritol
- ½ tsp onion powder
- ½ tsp garlic salt
- ½ tbsp dried parsley
- ½ tbsp baking powder
- ¼ tsp baking soda

Directions

1. Preheat now the waffle iron.
2. Meanwhile, in a bowl, whisk all the ingredients until smooth batter forms.
3. Open the iron, pour a quarter of the mixture into the iron, close and cook until crispy, 6 to 7 minutes.
4. Remove now the chaffle onto a plate and set aside.
5. Make three more Chaffles with the remaining batter.
6. Allow cooling and serve afterward.

Turnip Hash Brown Chaffles

Preparation: 10 minutes

Cooking: 42 minutes

Servings: 6

Ingredients

- 1 large turnip, peeled and shredded
- ½ medium white onion, minced
- 2 garlic cloves, pressed
- 1 cup finely grated Gouda cheese
- 2 eggs, beaten
- Salt and freshly ground black pepper to taste

Directions

1. Pour the turnips in a medium safe microwave bowl, sprinkle with 1 tbsp of water, and steam in the microwave until softened, 1 to 2 minutes.
2. Remove now the bowl and mix in the remaining ingredients except for a quarter cup of the Gouda cheese.
3. Preheat now the waffle iron.

4. Once heated, open and sprinkle some of the reserved cheese in the iron and top with 3 tbsps of the mixture. Close the waffle iron and cook until crispy, 5 minutes.
5. Open the lid, flip the chaffle and cook further for 2 more minutes.
6. Remove now the chaffle onto a plate and set aside.
7. Make five more chaffles with the remaining batter in the same proportion.
8. Allow cooling and serve afterward.

Everything Bagel Chaffles

Preparation: 10 minutes

Cooking: 28 minutes

Servings: 4

Ingredients

- 1 egg, beaten
- ½ cup finely grated Parmesan cheese
- 1 tsp Everything Bagel seasoning

Directions

1. Preheat now the waffle iron.
2. In a bowl, mix all the ingredients.
3. Open the iron, pour in a quarter of the mixture, close, and cook until crispy, 6 to 7 minutes.
4. Remove now the chaffle onto a plate and set aside.
5. Make three more chaffles, allow cooling, and enjoy after.

Blueberry Shortcake Chaffles

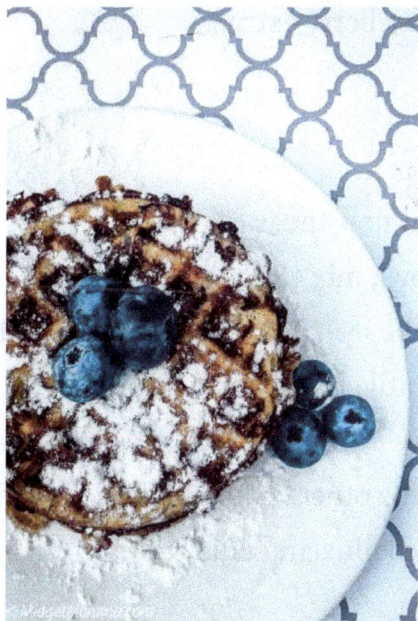

Preparation: 10 minutes

Cooking: 14 minutes

Servings: 2

Ingredients

- 1 egg, beaten
- 1 tbsp cream cheese, softened
- ¼ cup finely grated mozzarella cheese

- 1/4 tsp baking powder
- 4 fresh blueberries
- 1 tsp blueberry extract

Directions

1. Preheat now the waffle iron.
2. In a bowl, mix all the ingredients.
3. Open the iron, pour in half of the batter, close, and cook until crispy, 6 to 7 minutes.
4. Remove now the chaffle onto a plate and set aside.
5. Make the other chaffle with the remaining batter.
6. Allow cooling and enjoy after.

Raspberry-Pecan Chaffles

Preparation: 10 minutes

Cooking: 14 minutes

Servings: 2

Ingredients

- 1 egg, beaten
- ½ cup finely grated mozzarella cheese
- 1 tbsp cream cheese, softened
- 1 tbsp sugar-free maple syrup
- ¼ tsp raspberry extract
- ¼ tsp vanilla extract
- 2 tbsp sugar-free caramel sauce for topping
- 3 tbsp chopped pecans for topping

Directions

1. Preheat now the waffle iron.
2. In a bowl, mix all the ingredients.
3. Open the iron, pour in half of the batter, close, and cook until crispy, 6 to 7 minutes.
4. Remove now the chaffle onto a plate and set aside.

81

5. Make another chaffle with the remaining batter.
6. To serve: drizzle the caramel sauce on the chaffles and top with the pecans.

Breakfast Spinach Ricotta Chaffles

Preparation: 10 minutes

Cooking: 28 minutes

Servings: 4

Ingredients

- 4 oz frozen spinach, thawed, squeezed dry
- 1 cup ricotta cheese
- 2 eggs, beaten
- ½ tsp garlic powder
- ¼ cup finely grated Pecorino Romano cheese
- ½ cup finely grated mozzarella cheese
- Salt and freshly ground black pepper to taste

Directions

1. Preheat now the waffle iron.
2. In a bowl, mix all the ingredients.
3. Open the iron, lightly grease with cooking spray and spoon in a quarter of the mixture.
4. Close the iron and cook until brown and crispy, 7 minutes.
5. Remove now the chaffle onto a plate and set aside.

6. Make three more chaffles with the remaining mixture.
7. Allow cooling and serve afterward.

Scrambled Egg Stuffed Chaffles

Preparation: 15 minutes

Cooking: 28 minutes

Servings: 4

Ingredients

For the chaffles:

- 1 cup finely grated cheddar cheese
- 2 eggs, beaten

For the egg stuffing:

- 1 tbsp olive oil
- 4 large eggs
- 1 tiny green bell pepper, deseeded and chopped
- 1 tiny red bell pepper, deseeded and chopped
- Salt and freshly ground black pepper to taste
- 2 tbsp grated Parmesan cheese

Directions

For the chaffles:

1. Preheat now the waffle iron.

85

2. In a bowl, mix now the cheddar cheese and egg.

3. Open the iron, pour in a quarter of the mixture, close, and cook until crispy, 6 to 7 minutes.

4. Plate and make three more chaffles using the remaining mixture.

For the egg stuffing:

1. Meanwhile, heat the olive oil in a medium skillet over medium heat on a stovetop.

2. In a bowl, beat the eggs with the bell peppers, salt, black pepper, and Parmesan cheese.

3. Pour the mixture into the skillet and scramble until set to your likeness, 2 minutes.

4. Between two chaffles, spoon half of the scrambled eggs and Repeat now with the second set of chaffles.

5. Serve afterward.

Mixed Berry-Vanilla Chaffles

Preparation: 10 minutes

Cooking: 28 minutes

Servings: 4

Ingredients

- 1 egg, beaten
- ½ cup finely grated mozzarella cheese
- 1 tbsp cream cheese, softened
- 1 tbsp sugar-free maple syrup
- 2 strawberries, sliced
- 2 raspberries, slices
- ¼ tsp blackberry extract
- ¼ tsp vanilla extract
- ½ cup plain yogurt for serving

Directions

1. Preheat now the waffle iron.
2. In a bowl, mix all the ingredients except the yogurt.
3. Open the iron, lightly grease with cooking spray and pour in a quarter of the mixture.

4. Close the iron and cook until golden brown and crispy, 7 minutes.
5. Remove now the chaffle onto a plate and set aside.
6. Make three more chaffles with the remaining mixture.
7. To serve: top with the yogurt and enjoy.

Ham and Cheddar Chaffles

Preparation: 15 minutes

Cooking: 28 minutes

Servings: 4

Ingredients

- 1 cup finely shredded parsnips, steamed
- 8 oz ham, diced
- 2 eggs, beaten
- 1 ½ cups finely grated cheddar cheese
- ½ tsp garlic powder
- 2 tbsp chopped fresh parsley leaves
- ¼ tsp smoked paprika
- ½ tsp dried thyme
- Salt and freshly ground black pepper to taste

Directions

1. Preheat now the waffle iron.
2. In a bowl, mix all the ingredients.
3. Open the iron, lightly grease with cooking spray and pour in a quarter of the mixture.

4. Close the iron and cook until crispy, 7 minutes.

5. Remove now the chaffle onto a plate and set aside.

6. Make three more chaffles using the remaining mixture.

7. Serve afterward.

Chaffles With Strawberry Frosty

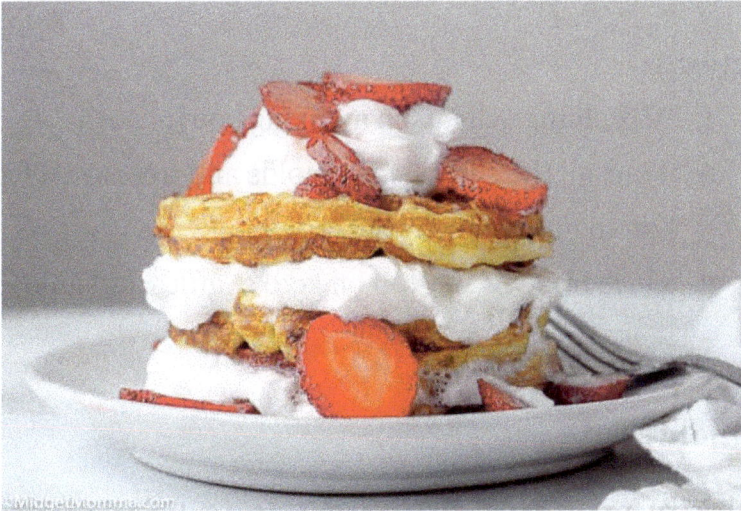

Preparation: 10 minutes

Cooking: 5 Minutes

Servings: 2

Ingredients

- 1 cup frozen strawberries
- 1/2 cup Heavy cream
- 1 tsp. stevia
- 1 scoop protein powder

91

- 3 keto chaffles (Choose a Recipes you like From Chapter 1)

Directions:

1. Mix all ingredients in a mixing bowl.
2. Pour mixture in silicone molds and freeze in a freezer for about 4 hours to set.
3. Once frosty is set, top on keto chaffles and enjoy!

Nutrition:

Carbohydrates: 9 g, Fats: 36 g, Proteins: 32 g, Calories: 474

Pecan Pumpkin Chaffle

Preparation: 20 minutes

Cooking: 15 Minutes

Servings: 2

Ingredients

- 1 egg
- 2 tbsp. pecans, toasted and chopped
- 2 tbsp. almond flour
- 1 tsp. erythritol
- 1/4 tsp. pumpkin pie spice
- 1 tbsp. pumpkin puree
- 1/2 cup Mozzarella cheese, grated

Directions

1. Preheat now your waffle maker.
2. Beat egg in a tiny bowl.
3. Add remaining ingredients and mix well.
4. Spray waffle maker with cooking spray.

5. Pour half batter in the hot waffle maker and cooking for minutes or until golden brown. Repeat now with the remaining batter.

6. Serve and enjoy.

Nutrition:

Calories: 240, Total Fat: 16 g, Protein: 21 g, Total Carbs: 3g, Fiber: 1g, Net Carbs: 2g

Bacon Chaffles With Herb Dip

Preparation: 6 minutes

Cooking: 10 Minutes

Servings: 2

Ingredients

Chaffles:

- 1 organic egg, beaten
- ½ cup Swiss/Gruyere cheese blend, shredded
- 2 tbsps cooked bacon pieces
- 1 tbspn jalapeño pepper, chopped

Dip:

- ¼ cup heavy cream
- ¼ teaspn fresh dill, minced
- Pinch of ground black pepper

Directions

1. Preheat now a mini waffle iron and then grease it.
2. For chaffles: In a bowl, put all ingredients and mix well.

3. Place half of the mixture into Preheat nowed waffle iron and cooking for about 5 minutes.

4. Repeat now with the remaining mixture.

5. Meanwhile, in a bowl, mix now the cream and stevia for dip.

6. Serve warm chaffles alongside the dip.

Nutrition:

Calories 147, Fat 14.2, Fiber 2.7, Carbs 6.1, Protein 1.4

Savory Gruyere and Chives Chaffles

Preparation: 15 minutes

Cooking: 14 minutes

Servings: 2

Ingredients

- 2 eggs, beaten
- 1 cup finely grated Gruyere cheese
- 2 tbsp finely grated cheddar cheese
- 1/8 tsp freshly ground black pepper
- 3 tbsp minced fresh chives + more for garnishing
- 2 sunshine fried eggs for topping

Directions

1. Preheat now the waffle iron.
2. In a bowl, mix now the eggs, cheeses, black pepper, and chives.
3. Open the iron and pour in half of the mixture.
4. Close the iron and cook until brown and crispy, 7 minutes.
5. Remove now the chaffle onto a plate and set aside.

6. Make another chaffle using the remaining mixture.
7. Top each chaffle with one fried egg each, garnish with the chives and serve.

Strawberry Shortcake Chaffle Bowls

Preparation: 15 minutes

Cooking: 28 Minutes

Servings: 2

Ingredients

- 1 egg, beaten
- ½ cup finely grated mozzarella cheese
- 1 tbsp almond flour
- ¼ tsp baking powder
- 2 drops cake batter extract
- 1 cup cream cheese, softened
- 1 cup fresh strawberries, sliced
- 1 tbsp sugar-free maple syrup

Directions

1. Preheat now a waffle bowl maker and grease lightly with cooking spray.
2. Meanwhile, in a bowl, whisk all the ingredients except the cream cheese and strawberries.

3. Open the iron, pour in half of the mixture, cover, and cook until crispy, 6 to 7 minutes.
4. Remove now the chaffle bowl onto a plate and set aside.
5. Make a second chaffle bowl with the remaining batter.
6. To serve, divide the cream cheese into the chaffle bowls and top with the strawberries.
7. Drizzle the filling with the maple syrup and serve.

Nutrition:

Calories 457, Total Fat 19.1 g, Saturated Fat 11 g, Cholesterol 262 mg, Total Carbs 8.9 g, Sugar 1.2 g, Fiber 1.7 g, Sodium 557 mg, Potassium 748 mg, Protein 32.5 g

Fluffy Sandwich Breakfast Chaffle

Preparation: 5 min

Cooking: 3 min

Servings: 2

Ingredients

- 1/2 tsp Psyllium husk powder (optional)
- tbsp almond flour
- 1/4 tsp Baking powder (optional)
- 1 large Egg
- 1/2 cup Mozzarella cheese, shredded
- 1 tbsp vanilla or
- Dash of cinnamon

Directions

1. Switch on your waffle maker according to manufacturer's Directions
2. Crack egg and combine with cheddar cheese in a tiny bowl
3. Add remaining ingredients and combine thoroughly.
4. Place half batter on waffle maker and spread evenly.

5. Cook for 4 minutes or until as desired
6. Gently Remove now from waffle maker and set aside for 2 minutes so it cools down and become crispy
7. Repeat for remaining batter
8. Serve with keto ice cream topping

Delicious Raspberries Taco Chaffles

Cooking: 15 Minutes

Servings: 1

Ingredients

- 1 egg white
- 1/4 cup jack cheese, shredded
- 1/4 cup cheddar cheese, shredded
- 1 tsp coconut flour
- 1/4 tsp baking powder
- 1/2 tsp stevia

For Topping:

- 4 oz. raspberries
- 2 tbsps. coconut flour
- 2 oz. unsweetened raspberry sauce

Directions

1. Switch on your round Waffle Maker and grease it with cooking spray once hot.
2. Mix all chaffle ingredients in a bowl and combine with a fork.

3. Pour chaffle batter in a Preheat nowed maker and close the lid.

4. Roll the taco chaffle around using a kitchen roller, set it aside and allow it to set for a few minutes.

5. Once the taco chaffle is set, Remove now from the roller.

6. Dip raspberries in sauce and arrange on taco chaffle.

7. Drizzle coconut flour on top.

8. Enjoy raspberries taco chaffle with keto coffee.

Nutrition:

Protein: 28% 77 kcal, Fat: 6 187 kcal, Carbohydrates: 3% 8 kcal

Chaffle Bruschetta

Cooking: 5 Minutes

Servings: 1

Ingredients

- 1/2 cup shredded mozzarella cheese
- 1 whole egg beaten
- 1/4 cup grated Parmesan cheese
- 1 tsp Italian Seasoning
- 1/4 tsp garlic powder

For the Toppings:

- 3-4 Cherry tomatoes, chopped
- 1 tsp fresh basil, chopped
- Splash of olive oil
- Pinch of salt

Directions

1. Turn on waffle maker to heat and oil it with cooking spray.
2. Whisk all chaffle ingredients except mozzarella, in a bowl.

3. Add in cheese and mix.

4. Add batter to waffle maker and cook for 5 minutes.

5. Mix tomatoes, basil, olive oil, and salt Serve over the top of chaffles.

Nutrition: Carbs: 2 g; Fat: 24 g; Calories: 352

Easter Morning Simple Chaffles

Cooking: 5 minutes

Servings: 2

Ingredients

- 1/2 cup egg whites
- 1 cup mozzarella cheese, Melt nowed

Directions

1. Switch on your square waffle maker. Spray with non-stick spray.
2. Beat egg whites with beater, until fluffy and white.
3. Add cheese and mix well.
4. Pour batter in a waffle maker.
5. Close the maker and cook for about 3 minutes.
6. Repeat now with the remaining batter.
7. Remove now chaffles from the maker.
8. Serve hot and enjoy!

Nutrition:

Protein: 36% 42 kcal, Fat: 60% 71kcal, Carbohydrates: 4% 5 kcal

Cheddar Protein Chaffles

Cooking: 40 Minutes

Servings: 8

Ingredients

- 1/2 cup golden flax seeds meal
- 1/2 cup almond flour
- 2 tbsps unsweetened whey protein powder
- 1 teaspn organic baking powder
- Salt and freshly ground black pepper to taste
- 3/4 cup Cheddar cheese, shredded
- 1/3 cup of unsweetened almond milk
- 2 tbsps unsalted butter, Melt nowed
- 2 large organic eggs, beaten

Directions

1. Preheat now a mini waffle iron and then grease It.
2. In a large bowl, place flax seeds meal, flour, protein powder, baking powder, and mix well.
3. Stir in the Cheddar cheese
4. In another bowl, place the remaining ingredients and beat until well combined.

5. Add the egg mixture into the bowl with flax seeds meal mixture and Mix well until well combined.
6. Place desired amount of the mixture into Preheat nowed waffle iron and cook for about 4-5 minutes or until golden brown.
7. Repeat now with the remaining mixture.
8. Serve warm.

www.ingramcontent.com/pod-product-compliance
Lightning Source LLC
Chambersburg PA
CBHW050754030426
42336CB00012B/1814